WHAT EVERY PERSON NEEDS TO KNOW ABOUT PEOPLE WITH DISABILITIES

Overcoming Attitudinal Barriers Towards People with Disabilities

by
Jessica Rodriguez

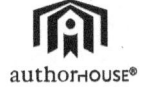
authorHOUSE®

AuthorHouse™
1663 Liberty Drive, Suite 200
Bloomington, IN 47403
www.authorhouse.com
Phone: 1-800-839-8640

First published by AuthorHouse 1/29/2008

ISBN: 978-1-4343-5419-8 (sc)

Printed in the United States of America
Bloomington, Indiana

This book is printed on acid-free paper.

DEDICATION

This book is dedicated to my mom and the rest of my family for giving me a chance in life. Thank you for the values that you've instilled in me. I love you and am eternally grateful. I also wish to dedicate this book to my Pastor and his wife Bishop Carlos and Mrs. Pamela Malone from Bethel Baptist Church. Thank you for mentoring me and for helping me grow spiritually and bringing out the gifts and talents God has given me. Thank you for loving me the way God loves and for seeing me not as Jess, the blind girl but as Jess, the person fearfully and wonderfuly made in the Image of God You have a special place in my heart.

ACKNOWLEDGMENTS

Thank you to my Lord and Savior Jesus Christ for sacrificing your life on the cross so I'd have eternal life.

Thanks to Jennifer and everyone at AuthorHouse for helping to make this book a success. Thank you to: Kammy, Alex, Janelle, Ken and Carmen. I'm blessed to have you as friends. Thank you to everyone at Bethel Full Gospel Baptist Church for embracing me as you have and for seeing me for who I am not for my disability.

TABLE OF CONTENTS

FOREWORD
BY MONIQUE LIGHTBOURNE—COATS

Silence is a crime as well as a tragedy in a time like ours when the lack of knowledge resonates in every sector of society. The shed blood of Jesus is the fullness of love expressed – God has plans for people with disabilities also.

As Jessica Rodriguez so eloquently proves, society tends to look at the outer being rather than the inner person. She has powerfully dispel the many myths and stereotypes that many have about people with disabilities. This is tall order!

However, the book you are about to read gives us fresh insight into this most misunderstood subject. Who can solve this? Jessica's wisdom is built on a life of realistic experiences. These experiences will hold up to the scrutiny of our culture.

This is a very important book in this hour in which we live. Read it until you over come attitudinal barriers about people with disabilities. The Spirit of God has inspired Jessica to bring this message to us and has anointed her to share parts of her life with us. As you explore this wisdom filled book, I know that you will join me in saying that God has indeed placed a mantle on Jessica that cannot be assumed by anyone and everyone, regardless of race, religion, nationality, gender, or socioeconomic status.

Despite her natural brilliance as a woman of God, Jessica is one of the most humble women I know. It is on the basis of her character and Christ-likeness that

I commend her to you. Your first line of defense will be to educate yourself by learning the truth that will bring you into freedom.

INTRODUCTION

The purpose of this book is to dispel the many myths and stereotypes that many have about people who have disabilities; be it a visual or hearing impairment or a physical or cognitive impairment. I pray that by sharing my experiences as someone with a visual impairment and sharing strategies to combat any attitude or intimidation you may have towards people with disabilities, you will soon see things in a different light.

CHAPTER 1:
GOD'S PLAN
DESPITE DISABILITY

Many ask if I'd rather be blind or wish to see. It's hard to say as I've never seen and feel blessed through this. There are many things in the world better left unseen, and I feel I have certain perspective that people who can see don't have. I don't get visually distracted by things around me and I don't consume myself with whether someone is fat, skinny, big or whatever. Being born blind and losing sight later in life each have good and bad aspects. When you've never seen, you don't miss seeing. Yet you have no concept of what things look like. When you lose sight later in life it's hard learning things in different ways, but you've seen so you have a reference point. Sit back and relax as we unravel the mystery and learn the secret to interacting with people who have disabilities.

Have you ever met someone who used a wheelchair or a cane? If so your first thought may have been, "Why does God allow people to be blind or need a wheelchair?" We'll never know the answer, but God does. I've been asked this question many times and some have said that I'm blind due to sin committed by my parents and that my blindness is a punishment. While we have all sinned and come short of the Glory of God, this idea is false and erroneous. This belief brings unnecessary and undeserved guilt on parents. There's a song that says "Jesus loves the little children, all the children of the world, red and yellow, black and white they are precious in his sight, Jesus loves the little children of the world." This holds true for children with disabilities. They need to be loved and held as any other child and not considered less due to their impairment.

There are many tests available today which can let future parents know whether their unborn child will have a disability such as Down Syndrome. This information should help prepare you, not scare you! I believe for any believer who may be going through this, your first line of defense should be to ask God for wisdom and strength to help you face whatever you may deal with. I've heard of people who choose to terminate pregnancy upon learning their baby has a disability. However, this is not the answer and is wrong in the eyes of God as you are killing a child which he created in his image. Exodus 4:11 reads, "who gave man his mouth and made him mute or deaf or blind? Is it not I the Lord?" God never gives more than we can handle. All children are gifts from God regardless of disability or not. A second line of defense for all parents of children with disabilities is a supportive family and church family. Many may say, "This doesn't affect me as I have no one in my family directly affected." This is the wrong mind set as we can all be affected at any time and we're not exempt as believers. In Jeremiah, the Lord says "I knew you before I formed you in your mother's womb." This means that before I ever existed, He knew I would be blind and though we may not understand, God has a purpose for everything and doesn't make mistakes. God uses anyone no matter how small the task may seem. As humans we may feel there is no hope, but Jeremiah 29:11 reads "for I know the plans I have for you plans to give you a hope and a future." We see despair but God gives hope.

While many have said my blindness is due to lack of faith, this could not be further from the truth. Someone asked if I believed God can heal me and make me whole. First, I am whole I just can't see, and secondly I believe that God can heal me if he chooses, but maybe there's a reason why He's allowed this. Prayer is powerful and that's the best thing you can do for someone with a disability besides giving love and support as you would anyone else.

Chapter 2:
Using People First Language: How to Address People with Disabilities

I recently went to the doctor with a family member and when they called me in, the medical assistant said to my companion, "Tell her to stand on the scale" as if I wasn't even there. Needless to say, it was an unpleasant experience! Let's look at ways to overcome this.

Words are very powerful and sometimes the things we say hurt more than physical wounds and can leave lasting scars. The Book of James talks about this and states that words can either give or take life. We don't realize it, but many times all of us, even the Body of Christ, tend to look at the outer being rather than the inner person. Samuel 1:16 says that "God looks at the heart while man looks at the outward appearance." I'm not saying that we shouldn't be well-groomed and present ourselves in a pleasant manner, but this is not what's most important. By solely looking at ones outer appearance, this brings division even among believers. I've heard it said that church is the most divided place there is because people only feel comfortable with their own kind. These things are not of God. While it's easy for me to say "I'm blind so I want to do activities for people with visual impairments or partake in social groups with those who are blind." I refuse to be put in a category. This is what we do when we label people. We should label things not people. Having stigmas and labels bring isolation and separation rather than unity.

Here are some words to avoid when referring to people with disability. Avoid words such as "handicap", "crippled", "retarded", "is a victim of" or "suffers from". These words bring negative connotations and are degrading to people. Although unintentional, many people use these terms not realizing the impact they have. Which statement sounds best? "My daughter is retarded" or "My daughter has an intellectual disability"? If you chose statement 2, you are correct as it puts the person first not the disability. Here are more examples of the right and wrong things to say. Don't say "My friend's in a wheelchair." Instead say "My friend uses a wheelchair." Say "I have a learning disability" not "I'm learning disabled." The wheelchair is the universal symbol for accessibility. Therefore, the hotel room is "wheelchair accessible" not "handicap accessible." Accessibility refers to the degree to which something is accessible. For instance a parking space is designated as "Accessible parking" with a permit, and not "Handicap parking." A person needing material in Braille uses the same materials a sighted person uses in an alternative or accessible format. A person with a hearing impairment may use an interpreter or an assistive listening device permitting them to hear clearly. By making these accommodations, you give people with disabilities equal access to the same information and facilities that other people have. This in turn achieves inclusion which brings respect and unity for all. Remember to use people first language and put the person first not the disability!

CHAPTER 3:
DISABILITY ETIQUETTES
DO'S AND DON'TS

Have you ever had someone move your belongings without your permission or give out your number without asking? I've had this happen and I want to be given the same respect that anyone else receives. Here are some things to smooth out the rough edges. Etiquette refers to how to treat people with consideration. While it seems obvious, many lack this regarding people with some kind of impairment. First, treat others as you'd like to be treated. I'd say the number one complaint of people with all types of disabilities is "people talk to my partner rather than to me." Always speak to the person directly not through a third party. How would you feel if someone spoke to your spouse asking what you wanted to drink instead of asking you directly? When working with interpreters for those with hearing impairments, speak to the person not the interpreter. Remember people with disabilities are humans and by talking to a partner rather than the person, it is as if they don't exist. Treat them with the same respect that you wish to be given. People with disabilities are individuals with their own unique God given talents and personalities. Never compare one to another. Ask for permission to give them a hug as you would anyone else as not everyone likes being touched. Respect their desire to make decisions and do things for themselves. For many people with disabilities, it's easy for those around you to want to dictate what to do, where to go or even who they feel you should marry. Only God knows these things. By saying to someone, "can I get that for you?" You're trying to be helpful but in actuality, you're taking control of the situation. It's best to give the person a chance to do something on their own and if help is needed, they'll ask. Don't assume someone is unable due to their impairment. Respect someone's belongings and don't move or touch it without asking. Don't give out their phone number with out asking. Again, this sounds obvious, but these things have happened to me before. It's ok to do nice things for someone, but if a man orders my meal, would he do this for all the ladies or is he doing it because he thinks I can't due to my visual impairment. That's what people need to separate or differentiate. If you ask to help someone and your help is refused, don't be offended just let them do it on their own. Doing everything for someone doesn't help; it harms them and doesn't give them a sense of independence. It may take someone a little longer but in the end, they'll celebrate knowing they were able to do it on their own in your absence. This doesn't mean you are not needed, but it means there are other ways you can provide support.

CHAPTER 4:
HOW THE BODY OF CHRIST CAN SUPPORT PEOPLE WITH DISABILITIES AND THEIR FAMILIES

My Pastor, Bishop Carlos L. Malone Senior, has a way with people and is unique in many ways. Some time ago, we were given a quiz in Bible study. Rather than ignoring the situation and not giving me the test at all, he assigned one of my classmates to read the test and fill in my answers. He chose to work around the situation rather than avoiding it and has always made me feel that I have much to offer at Bethel.

While God is the only one who can meet all of our needs, he did create us to have relationship with each other and we are all interdependent. We all need relationships: friends to love and be loved by, people who will pray with us, or someone to talk to when struggling. Due to lack of knowledge and understanding, many churches don't know how to provide support because it's something unknown. Rather than facing it head on, they shy away and say, "We don't know how to deal with your impairment" or "here's a ministry for people with disabilities." I read about a church who wanted to adopt people with Down Syndrome. Instead of including them at the dinner table with other congregation members, they seated these individuals in a corner alone. That's not inclusion, that's exclusion! Maybe they had the best of intentions, but because they didn't take time to learn about Down Syndrome and the different ways of dealing with it, they sent a message of rejection rather than love and acceptance.

Here are some tips to make you more at ease. First, give family members and the person with a disability the freedom and opportunity to express how they feel. Emotional support is important for all of us. At times we just need someone to listen while we share; we are not necessarily looking for a solution or quick fix. Sometimes you don't need to say anything; just listen and put your arm around them. Maybe a mom has a child with autism and needs a break; offer to take the child to the park. Maybe the church is going on a trip to the zoo and you have a member using a wheelchair. Assign people to take turns pushing the chair if required. Maybe someone has lost their sight and has trouble adjusting. Focus on their abilities and help them in their training process by offering to walk around the block along side them as they learn to use their cane. These are small ways in which the Body of Christ can give support. By doing so, you'll not only build a relationship and help someone, but they will also help you and bless your life.

CHAPTER 5:
TIPS FOR WORKING WITH PEOPLE WHO HAVING VISUAL IMPAIRMENTS

One of the most uncomfortable things for someone who is visually impaired is being in a room full of people and not knowing who is around. In this chapter you will learn how to deal with this and many other situations you may encounter when dealing with someone with a visual impairment.

Always identify yourself when entering and exiting a room and introduce all parties in the room. Just because someone has some vision doesn't mean they know where you are or who you are. Give your name so the person can connect a name with your voice. Seventy-five percent of communication is nonverbal, but this doesn't work with someone who has a visual impairment. You may smile at someone or wink to show you care but for people with vision problems, particularly who are totally blind, you need to communicate with your voice. If you want to convey "I'm happy to see you" let this reflect in your voice. Instead of winking or waving, shake their hand. Gestures and facial expressions won't help the person much if they can't see. When in conversation, be an active listener; remember they can't see you so say "I understand" or "I see." They need to know you're listening, not reading the paper. When in a group of people, always address whom you're talking to so the person won't be confused and think you're talking to them when you're not. When in a conversation, let the person know you're stepping out a second so they don't talk to an empty chair as this is embarrassing. Don't be afraid of using words like, "See you later" or "Did you watch the movie?" These are every day words and should not be avoided just as we shouldn't avoid words about hearing or running because someone has mobility impairment or hearing impairment.

Describe to the person with a visual impairment what's going on around them and talk about colors shapes or patterns. Don't alter anything; just be to the point. Say the kids are in blue jeans and white shirts and are dancing. Someone who can't see has no idea about the world around them unless you teach them and describe things. You see and take in information visually, but for someone who can't you may need to have them touch a football to understand a concept or experience a baseball game to understand. Don't assume because someone can't see they shouldn't go to a ballet or go shopping. They can't see the clothes but can feel the material and you can tell them what color goes with what and what can be washed and can't. We all want to know our surroundings right? So do people who can't see. Always describe the room using the door as a reference point. Say, "The door is behind you and we're in a big circle shaped room with bikes where people work out." Walk the person around and let them touch objects around them if needed. Always explain things in relation to the person's body. The door is to your left or John's in front of you. You can also use the clock face and say "The sink's at 3 and the soap at 5." Also use this method when describing location of food on a plate.

When guiding someone, use the "sighted guide" techniques. The following will make walking safe and comfortable for all. Never grab their arm or steer the person. Tap their hand with the back of your hand signifying to take your arm so you need not tell them to do so. Be sure the follower is always a half step behind you and slightly to the side ensuring they feel your movements and cues. Relax your arm at your side and walk normally. You need not indicate "left turn, right turn" as they'll feel your body movement. When approaching narrow spaces, move your arm diagonally across your back and the person will get behind you in single file and slide their hand down to your wrist. Again, you need not say anything as they'll know the cue. When the area widens, move your guiding arm forward and the person holds above your elbow again. When turning around, tell the person you need to turn and stop walking and both parties will do an about face then resume position. When approaching stairs and curbs, briefly pause before stepping up or down so the person can catch up to you. You need not say up down or count steps as they feel your movements. If you must separate briefly, place their hand on a wall, counter, chair or some kind of object so they don't lose orientation and never leave them in free space. When approaching doors, indicate verbally if it's a pull or push door. Open the door and indicate which side the door's on and if it faces towards or away from them. Then let them hold the door as you walk through. When guiding to a chair, place their hand on the back of the chair and let them seat themselves.

CHAPTER 6:
ADVICE FOR PARENTS

I remember reading about a lady whose daughter was blind so she decided to learn Braille and help her daughter with her homework and was actively involved in her daughter's life.

To all parents with children or adults with disabilities, my first piece of advice is to check your attitude as it determines whether your child makes it or breaks it. Do you have expectations for your child that all parents have for their kids to get an education, marry and have a family? Do you see him or her as a person who has much to offer or do you see them as someone needing to be hidden from the world. How you feel and deal with his or her disability will greatly impact how he or she feels about himself. I'd encourage you to help them lead the most normal life possible and give them the same unconditional love and support you'd give your children without disabilities. Encourage them to dream big and establish friendships based on interests, character and morality rather than disability. Don't put your child in a category but love them with the love that God loves. Model acceptance in your home and teach their friends that although your child has a disability, he and his friends have more similarities than differences. Don't focus on what they can't do rather focus on what they can. So many parents say, "We knew there was something wrong when" or "My son can't play ball like the other kids." He may not play ball but find something he can do.

This kind of negative talk messes people up and doesn't help self-image. Treat and love your child as the precious child given from God not as your child with a disability. Yes, you should realize his or her limitations, but we all have limitations and disabilities. Sometimes, emotional hang ups or insecurities are more damaging or crippling than physical disabilities. I believe that spiritual blindness is far worse than physical blindness. Encourage them to make decisions and, yes, they'll make mistakes but love them through it. We all make mistakes and will all fail. That is part of life. But does God stop loving us when we fail? I don't think so. Just as God keeps supporting us, so should parents do the same for their children even those with disabilities.

Chapter 7:
"To Marry or not to Marry; That is the Question"

In second grade my teacher, Ms. Louder Milk, invited us to her wedding. I remember feeling her veil and her beautiful white dress. Sometime later, she was pregnant and I felt the baby kicking in her big belly. I remember thinking, "When I grow up, I want to marry and have a baby inside just like her. I imagined wearing my veil and carrying a baby inside me. I wasn't old enough to know what I wanted in a potential mate, but knew that's what I wanted when I grew up.

Ms. Louder Milk taught me about persistence and always told me "when you fall, you have to pick yourself up and keep going." To all the married people, I'm sure you remember your single days. Oh how you desired to date and imagined what your future mate would be like. You remember going on your first date, the first time you held hands and the friendship you formed which led to your marriage. Then you felt the excitement of planning the wedding and making all of those invitations ensuring everything was perfect. Then you found out you were expecting a year after your wedding, and this too, brought more excitement! Single people have these same aspirations including those with disabilities. The problem lies in the fact that people perceive that because someone has a disability they should marry someone with a disability as well because that person will understand how they feel. This isn't always true. There are people with disabilities who are mean, bitter and have no empathy whatsoever. Secondly, you don't base a relationship of any kind be it a friendship or marriage on someone's skin color or disability. You need to look at the person's character. Are they following Christ? Is this person a Christian? Do you share the same values and principles? Are they moral and honest? Do they have a stable job? How do they treat their family? Whether a person is blind or not is irrelevant. You love someone for who they are not for what they can or can't do. People will never fully understand what the other person goes through, but does that mean that they can't have a relationship and try to understand and empathize with each other? Many have told me that I'd be a burden on my future spouse and that he would want someone who isn't limited by their mobility, someone who is independent. It all has to do with mind set. Will he choose to see me as a precious woman given by God or will he focus on the fact that I can't see and will require assistance in certain areas. Will he choose to see my qualities and the things I can offer in the relationship or will he focus on what I can't do? Every relationship requires time and commitment and all relationships pose challenges regardless of disability or not. Will being married to someone with a disability pose different challenges? Yes, but will you look beyond that and overcome it together or will you choose to look the other way?

I'm reminded of Christopher Reeves and his wife Dayna. It was such a beautiful story of love and devotion. Dayna said that after her husband became paralyzed, this brought them much closer. I'm sure it would have been easier for her to say to him, "Sweet-heart, I want a divorce because you're not the way you use to be." Instead, she stuck by him and although he couldn't care for himself and needed help dressing and feeding, to her, he was still her husband not someone in a wheelchair. This is a story of true love and sacrifice. As mentioned earlier, we all need each other and need help as no one is an island. Women who give birth need their husbands to help with cleaning and cooking sometimes as they recover from having a baby and getting up every 3-4 hours. Is the fact that I may need my future partner to read the mail or read the cooking instructions so burdensome? There are many things I can do for him also. Where's the love and commitment that Christ teaches about and do we really try to practice this in the Body of Christ? Marriage and intimacy is something God created and everyone should have the right to experience that, even those with disabilities.

CHAPTER 8:
WHAT'S NEXT?

To sum things up, the best thing I could say is when you encounter someone with a disability, try to get to know them as you would anyone else. Just relax and be yourself. Start a dialog asking where they're from or what they do for a living. If you're not yet comfortable, I encourage you to find someone with a disability and have lunch together. Try to get to know them in various settings such as a restaurant or at a movie. Knowing someone at church or talking for 5 minutes after service doesn't cut it. This applies to people with and without disabilities. It takes time and effort, but time is something you make not something you have. If you are really interested in pursuing a relationship, you'll invest in that person and that person will invest in you. In the end, it's a win-win situation and all will be blessed.

Resources

Here are some helpful resources

The American Foundation for the blind:
www.afb.org

The Muscular Dystraphy Association:
www.mda.org

The Epilepsy Foundation:
www.epilepsyfoundation.org

Best Buddies: www.bestbuddies.org

Autism Society of America:
www.autism-society.org

The Down Syndrome Foundation:
www.downsyndromefoundation.org.

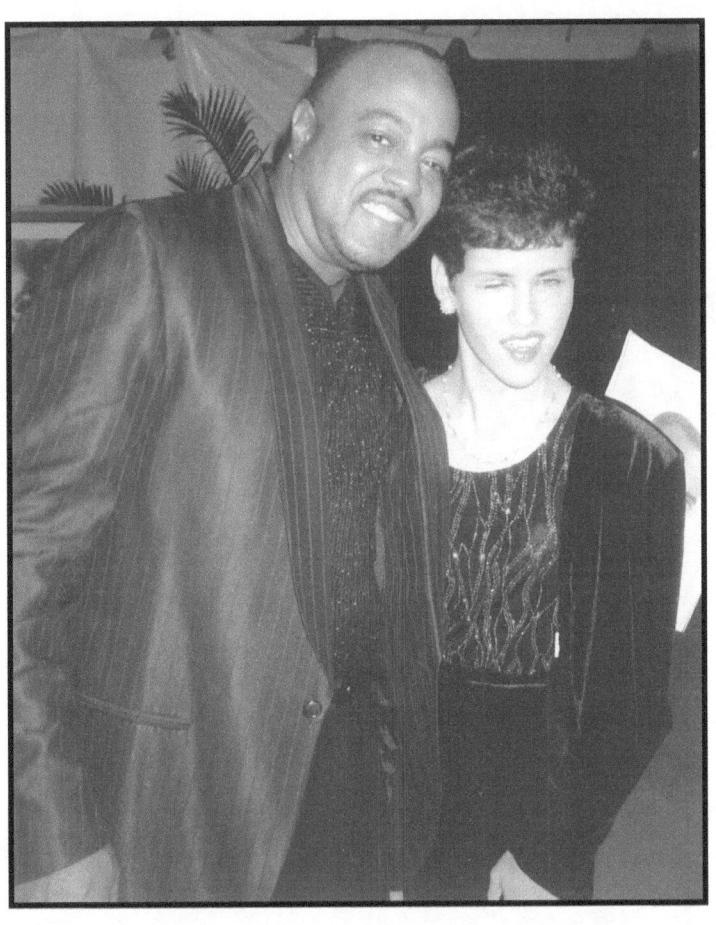

The author, Jessica Rodriguez, with Oscar-winning singer Peabo Bryson.